Menopause and Diversity:

Exploring the Impact of Race and Ethnicity on Women's Health

Copyright @Menopause Matter 2023
ISBN : 978-1-7389796-0-8
Author @Gillianne Fuller
Publisher @COJ BOOKZ
Book Cover @Samful Ueller
Edited @Heather Desna
Formatted @Samiahmed321
Contact @info@menopausematter.org
Website @ www.menopausematter.org
Website @ www.menopausematter.ca

Dedication

We would like to dedicate this book to all those who have supported our organization, Menopause Matter. To those who have generously donated their time and resources to help us further our mission of providing women with the knowledge and support they need to manage their menopause journey with confidence and ease.

We would like to thank our donors, whose contributions have allowed us to continue our important work, and those who have purchased this book, helping us to raise awareness and provide resources to women across the globe. We are grateful for the unwavering support of our partners, volunteers, and staff, whose tireless efforts have helped us to make a positive impact in the lives of so many women.

To all the women who have shared their stories and experiences with us, we thank you. Your courage and honesty have helped us to create a community of support and understanding, where women can come together to learn, share, and grow.

Finally, we dedicate this book to all women who are navigating their menopause journey. We hope that the information and resources contained within these pages will help you to feel empowered, informed, and confident as you navigate this important life stage.

Thank you for your support of Menopause Matter, and for your commitment to the health and well-being of women everywhere.

Menopause and Diversity:

Table Of Contents

INTRODUCTION v

Black Women and Menopause 1

Asian Women and Menopause...23

Indigenous Women and Menopause 34

Socioeconomic Status and Menopause 43

SUMMARY 46

REFERENCES..47

INTRODUCTION

INTRODUCTION

Menopause is a natural and inevitable part of every woman's life, but its impact can vary widely depending on factors such as age, health status, and lifestyle. Additionally, emerging research has highlighted the importance of considering the impact of race and ethnicity on menopausal experiences, as women from different racial and ethnic backgrounds may experience menopause in distinct ways. This book seeks to delve into the ways in which menopause affects women from different racial and ethnic backgrounds, exploring the unique challenges and opportunities presented by these diverse experiences. By highlighting some of the differences, this book aims to foster greater understanding and compassion around menopause, and to promote more inclusive and culturally sensitive approaches to women's health.

Black, Asian, and Latina women on average begin menopause earlier than white women. Non-Hispanic white women's average age at final menstrual period (FMP) was 51.4 years; Latina women from the New York–New Jersey area had theirs 1.7 years earlier, Chinese women from Oakland 1.2 years earlier, and Black women from Pittsburgh, Detroit, and Boston 1.2 years earlier.

Some groups experience the symptoms associated with menopause even late into the transition. The average duration

Menopause and Diversity:

of menopause-related hot flashes and night sweats was 6.5 years in non-Hispanic white women, 8.9 years in Latina women, and 10.1 years in Black women. Lean Black women — as opposed to Black women with obesity — are most likely to have the longest lasting and most severe hot flashes. On the flip side, in Chinese American women they lasted 5.4 years, and in Japanese American women from Los Angeles they lasted 4.8 years.

Latina women have more complaints of vaginal symptoms, **vaginal dryness** and painful sex, and interestingly vaginal symptoms vary by sub-ethnicity, in that Central American and South American Hispanic women (compared with Caribbean Hispanic women) reported having the worst symptoms.

Some studies show that Native American women had more hot flashes than any ethnic group in their thirties and forties prior to menopause and some studies implies that Native American women may have the very worst menopausal experience.

Black Women and Menopause

Research has shown that African American women tend to have more severe symptoms of menopause, such as hot flashes, night sweats, and sleep disturbances, compared to women of other racial and ethnic groups. They may also experience these symptoms for a longer period. 46% of Black women, compared to 37% of white women, reported experiencing hot flashes and 27% of Black women reported clinically significant depressive symptoms, whilst only 22% white women reported the same symptom.

To expand on this, it's important to note that the reasons behind these differences are not fully understood. However, some possible explanations have been suggested. For example, some researchers have hypothesized that genetic factors may play a role in the severity of menopausal symptoms experienced by African American women. Other factors, such as differences in lifestyle or environmental exposures, may also contribute.

Hot flashes:

Hot flashes are a common symptom of menopause that can involve sudden feelings of heat in the upper body, flushing, and sweating. Some studies have found that Black women tend to have more severe hot flashes than women of other races and ethnicities. In addition, Black women may experience hot flashes for a longer period, with some studies suggesting that the average duration of hot flashes in Black women is around 11 years.

Studies have found that variations in certain genes that are involved in regulating body temperature and responding to stress may be more common in Black women, which could make them more vulnerable to hot flashes and other menopausal symptoms.

Another factor is lifestyle and environmental factors. Black women may be more likely to live in hotter climates, which can contribute to feeling overheated and increase the frequency and intensity of hot flashes. Additionally, some cultural practices, such as wearing protective hairstyles or clothing that can trap heat, may also contribute to feelings of warmth and contribute to hot flashes.

Finally, Black women may also be more likely to experience higher levels of stress and anxiety due to racism and discrimination, which can contribute to dysregulation of the body's stress response and exacerbate hot flashes and other menopausal symptoms.

It's important to note that the experience of menopause is unique to each individual, and not all Black women will necessarily experience more severe or longer-lasting hot flashes. It's essential for each person to discuss their individual health concerns and needs with their healthcare provider to develop a personalized treatment plan that meets their unique needs.

Night sweats:

Night sweats, which involve sweating and flushing during sleep, are also a common symptom of menopause. Black women may experience more severe night sweats than women of other races and ethnicities, which can contribute to sleep disturbances and fatigue.

Black women may be particularly vulnerable to night sweats during menopause due to various social and cultural factors, such as living in hotter climates, wearing protective hairstyles or clothing that can contribute to feeling overheated, and experiencing higher levels of stress and anxiety due to racism and discrimination.

Night sweats can be particularly disruptive to sleep, leading to feelings of fatigue, irritability, and difficulties with concentration and memory. They can also contribute to feelings of embarrassment or shame.

To manage night sweats during menopause, Black women can try various strategies, such as wearing lightweight and breathable clothing to bed, using fans or air conditioning to keep the bedroom cool, and avoiding spicy or hot foods that can contribute to feeling overheated. Engaging in relaxation techniques such as meditation, yoga, or deep breathing exercises may also help promote feelings of relaxation and reduce the likelihood of night sweats.

Sleep disturbances:

Sleep disturbances are a common symptom of menopause and can include difficulty falling asleep or staying asleep, as well as waking up feeling tired. Black women may be more likely to experience sleep disturbances during menopause, which can have a negative impact on overall health and well-being.

Due to social and cultural factors such as experiences of racism and discrimination, which can contribute to stress and anxiety that interfere with sleep. Additionally, factors such as financial stress, caregiving responsibilities, and work-related stress may also contribute to sleep difficulties among Black women.

Sleep disturbances during menopause can take several forms, including difficulty falling asleep, waking up frequently during the night, and waking up too early in the morning. These disruptions can lead to fatigue, irritability, and difficulties with concentration and memory.

There are several strategies that can help Black women manage sleep disturbances during menopause. These may include practicing good sleep hygiene, such as establishing a consistent bedtime routine and creating a comfortable sleep environment. Avoiding stimulants such as caffeine and nicotine, especially in the evening, can also be helpful. Additionally, engaging in relaxation techniques such as meditation, yoga, or deep breathing exercises can promote feelings of relaxation and help prepare the body for sleep.

For women who are experiencing significant sleep disturbances or insomnia, working with a healthcare provider to develop a treatment plan may be necessary. This may involve medications or other interventions to help regulate sleep, such as cognitive-behavioral therapy for insomnia (CBT-I).

Mood changes:

Menopause can also be associated with mood changes, such as irritability, anxiety, and depression. Black women may be more likely to experience these mood changes during menopause, which can be related to a range of social, cultural, and environmental factors. For Black women, there may be additional social and cultural factors that impact mood changes during menopause. These can include experiences of racism and discrimination, which can lead to increased stress and anxiety, as well as cultural expectations around strength and resilience that may make it difficult to express vulnerability or seek help for emotional struggles.

In addition, Black women may be more likely to have certain underlying health conditions, such as hypertension, which can contribute to more severe menopausal symptoms. Menopause can have a range of effects on a Black woman's health beyond the common symptoms such as hot flashes, night sweats, and sleep disturbances. Here are a few additional examples:

Cardiovascular health:

Menopause can increase a woman's risk for cardiovascular disease. This is particularly true for Black women, who are already at a higher risk for heart disease due to factors such as hypertension, diabetes, and obesity. During menopause, women may experience changes in their cholesterol levels and blood pressure, which can contribute to a higher risk of heart disease. Cardiovascular disease is a major health concern for Black women, and menopause can further increase the risk of heart disease.

Here are a few key points to consider:

Risk factors:

Black women are at a higher risk of developing cardiovascular disease compared to women of other races and ethnicities. Risk factors for heart disease include high blood pressure, high cholesterol, obesity, and diabetes, all of which are more common among Black women. During menopause, women may experience changes in their blood pressure and cholesterol levels, which can further increase their risk of heart disease.

Hormonal changes:

The decline in estrogen levels during menopause may also contribute to changes in the cardiovascular system. Estrogen helps protect the heart by relaxing blood vessels and reducing inflammation, and the loss of this protective effect may increase the risk of heart disease.

Lifestyle factors:

Lifestyle factors such as diet, exercise, and smoking can also contribute to cardiovascular health. Black women may be more likely to consume diets high in sodium and saturated fat, which can increase blood pressure and cholesterol levels. Additionally, Black women may be less likely to engage in regular physical activity, which can help reduce the risk of heart disease. Smoking is also a significant risk factor for heart disease, and Black women may be more likely to smoke compared to women of other races and ethnicities.

Access to care:

Black women may face barriers to accessing healthcare, which can impact their cardiovascular health. These barriers may include lack of insurance, limited availability of healthcare providers, and discrimination in the healthcare system.

Overall, it's important for Black women to be aware of their risk of cardiovascular disease and to take steps to reduce their risk. This may include managing other health conditions such as hypertension and diabetes, making lifestyle changes such as improving their diet and increasing physical activity, and discussing their cardiovascular risk with their healthcare provider.

Bone health:

Menopause can also affect a woman's bone health, leading to a higher risk of osteoporosis and bone fractures. This risk is particularly high for Black women, who have lower bone density on average than women of other races and ethnicities.

Menopause and Diversity:

There are several factors that may contribute to lower bone density in Black women compared to women of other races and ethnicities.

Here are a few possibilities:

Genetics: Bone density is partly determined by genetics, and some studies suggest that there may be genetic differences in bone density among different racial and ethnic groups. For example, some studies have identified certain genes that are more common in Black individuals and may be associated with lower bone density.

Hormonal factors:

Hormones such as estrogen and testosterone play a key role in maintaining bone density, and hormonal changes during menopause can contribute to bone loss. Black women may have lower levels of estrogen on average, which could make them more vulnerable to bone loss.

Lifestyle factors:

Lifestyle factors such as diet and exercise can also affect bone density. Black women may be more likely to consume diets that are low in calcium and vitamin D, which are important for bone health. Additionally, Black women may be less likely to engage in weight-bearing exercise, which can help build and maintain bone density.

Other health conditions:

Black women are also more likely to have health conditions that can contribute to bone loss, such as hypertension, diabetes, and obesity. These conditions can affect bone density directly or indirectly, through their impact on hormone levels, inflammation, and other processes.

It's important to note that the reasons for lower bone density in Black women are not fully understood, and more research is needed to identify the underlying factors and develop effective interventions. However, it's clear that Black women may be at increased risk of osteoporosis and fractures during menopause and should be screened regularly for bone density.

Sexual health:

Menopause can also affect a woman's sexual health, leading to changes in libido, vaginal dryness, and discomfort during sex. Black women may be particularly reluctant to discuss these issues with healthcare providers, which can lead to underdiagnosis and undertreatment of sexual health problems during menopause.

Here are a few points to consider:

Vaginal dryness:

As estrogen levels decline during menopause, many women experience vaginal dryness, which can cause discomfort and pain during sex. Black women may be more likely to experience vaginal dryness due to lower estrogen levels on average, which can have a negative impact on sexual function and quality of life.

Changes in libido:

Some women may also experience changes in libido or sexual desire during menopause, which can be related to hormonal changes or other factors such as stress, depression, or relationship issues.

Pelvic floor dysfunction:

Menopause can also contribute to pelvic floor dysfunction, which can cause urinary incontinence, vaginal prolapse, and other issues that can impact sexual function and quality of life.

Cultural and social factors:

Cultural and social factors may also play a role in sexual health and function among Black women. For example, stigma around sexuality and lack of access to sexual health information and resources may contribute to sexual health disparities.

It's important for Black women to discuss any changes in sexual health or function with their healthcare provider, who can offer guidance and treatment options. Treatment options may include vaginal moisturizers or lubricants, hormone therapy, pelvic floor exercises, or other interventions as appropriate. It's also important to address any cultural or social factors that may impact sexual health and function, and to seek out resources and support as needed.

Mental health:

Menopause can also have an impact on a woman's mental health, increasing the risk of depression, anxiety, and other mood disorders. Black women may be particularly vulnerable to mental health problems during menopause due to a range of social and cultural factors, such as discrimination, stress, and trauma.

Here are a few key points to consider:

Mood changes:

Many women experience mood changes during menopause, which can include symptoms such as irritability, anxiety, depression, and mood swings. These symptoms may be related to hormonal changes during menopause, as well as other factors such as stress, sleep disturbances, and chronic health conditions.

Stigma and cultural factors:

Stigma and cultural factors may also contribute to mental health disparities among Black women. For example, Black women may face barriers to accessing mental health care, including lack of insurance or healthcare providers, stigma around mental health, and cultural norms around seeking help.

Coping strategies:

Coping strategies can also play a role in mental health during menopause. Black women may be more likely to rely on social support networks and community resources, which can be important sources of resilience and strength during times of stress.

Hormone therapy:

Hormone therapy may also have an impact on mental health during menopause. Some studies have suggested that hormone therapy may improve mood and reduce symptoms of depression and anxiety in some women, although the risks and benefits of this treatment should be carefully considered on an individual basis.

It's important for Black women to discuss any concerns about mental health with their healthcare provider, who can offer guidance and treatment options. This may include counseling, medication, lifestyle changes, or other interventions as appropriate. It's also important to address any cultural or social factors that may impact mental health, and to seek out resources and support as needed.

Black women may be more likely to experience early menopause.

Early menopause, which is defined as menopause occurring before the age of 40, is less common among all women, including Black women. However, some studies have suggested that Black women may be at higher risk for early menopause compared to women of other racial and ethnic backgrounds.

There are several factors that may contribute to this increased risk. One factor is genetics. Black women have been found to have a higher prevalence of genetic variations that are associated with early menopause, such as mutations in the BRCA1 and BRCA2 genes. Additionally, some studies have suggested that Black women may have lower levels of anti-Mullerian hormone (AMH), which is a hormone that is used as a marker of ovarian reserve and can impact the timing of menopause.

Other factors that may contribute to early menopause among Black women include exposure to environmental toxins, autoimmune disorders, and lifestyle factors such as smoking and excessive alcohol consumption.

Early menopause can have significant health impacts for Black women, including an increased risk of osteoporosis, cardiovascular disease, and cognitive decline. It can also impact fertility and emotional well-being.

Given the potential health impacts of early menopause, it's important for Black women who experience symptoms of menopause before the age of 40 to seek out medical attention and support. This may involve working with a healthcare provider to develop a plan for managing symptoms and reducing long-term health risks, as well as seeking out emotional support from family, friends, or mental health professionals.

Menopause and Diversity:

Black women may be less likely to receive appropriate care for menopausal symptoms.

Despite the higher prevalence of menopausal symptoms in Black women, they may be less likely to receive appropriate care for these symptoms. This may be due to a range of factors, including systemic racism and bias within the healthcare system, as well as cultural attitudes towards menopause.

Cultural attitudes towards menopause may play a role in the experience of menopause among Black women.

In some Black communities, menopause may be viewed as a taboo subject, which can lead to a lack of knowledge and understanding about the process. This can contribute to a lack of appropriate care and support for women going through menopause. However, it's important to note that attitudes towards menopause can vary widely within and between different Black communities as experiences and beliefs are shaped by a range of factors such as religion, region, and family background.

One attitude that has been noted among some Black women is a reluctance to discuss menopause openly. Menopause may be viewed as a private or personal matter, and some women may feel uncomfortable discussing it with others. There may also be a sense of shame or stigma around menopause, particularly around symptoms such as hot flashes or vaginal dryness.

On the other hand, some Black women may view menopause as a natural and expected part of the aging process. Menopause may be seen as a time to focus on personal growth and reflection, and to prioritize self-care and well-being. Some women may also view menopause as a time of increased wisdom and maturity and may seek out supportive networks of other women going through menopause.

Overall, cultural attitudes towards menopause are complex and can vary widely among Black women. It's important to recognize and respect individual experiences and beliefs, and to provide support and resources that are tailored to each woman's unique needs and preferences.

Social support can be an important factor in managing menopausal symptoms.

Social support, such as having access to a supportive partner or community, can be an important factor in managing the symptoms of menopause. Black women may face unique challenges in accessing social support, due to a range of factors such as systemic racism and social isolation.

There are several social, economic, and other factors that may affect Black women in menopause, including:

Lack of access to healthcare:

Black women may face barriers to accessing healthcare, including lack of insurance or healthcare providers, which can impact their ability to receive adequate care during menopause.

Racial and gender discrimination:

Black women may also face discrimination and bias in healthcare settings, which can impact the quality of care they receive and their ability to advocate for their health needs

Socioeconomic factors:

Black women are more likely to experience poverty, unemployment, and other socioeconomic challenges, which can impact their access to healthcare, nutrition, and other resources that can support their health during menopause

Cultural factors:

Cultural factors may also impact the experience of menopause in Black women. For example, stigma and shame around aging and menopause may contribute to a lack of discussion and awareness around menopause in some Black communities.

Family responsibilities:

Black women may also be more likely to be caregivers for children, grandchildren, and elderly family members, which can impact their ability to prioritize their own health needs during menopause.

Lack of social support:

Black women may also face challenges in accessing social support networks, which can be important sources of emotional and practical support during menopause.

Work-related stress:

Black women may also experience higher levels of work-related stress and discrimination, which can impact their overall health and well-being during menopause.

Here are some things that black women can do to help manage their menopause symptoms:

Talk to a healthcare provider:

Black women should talk to their healthcare provider about their menopause symptoms and any concerns they may have. This can help them get a proper diagnosis and treatment plan.

Exercise regularly:

Regular exercise can help improve mood, sleep quality, and overall health. Black women should aim to get at least 30 minutes of moderate intensity exercise most days of the week. Here are some types of exercise that may be particularly helpful:

Aerobic exercise: Aerobic exercise, such as brisk walking, jogging, cycling, or dancing, can help improve cardiovascular health, manage weight, and reduce the risk of chronic diseases such as diabetes and heart disease.

Strength training: Strength training, such as lifting weights or using resistance bands, can help maintain muscle mass and bone density, both of which can decline during menopause.

Yoga or stretching: Yoga or stretching can help improve flexibility, balance, and posture, as well as reduce stress and improve mood.

High-intensity interval training (HIIT): HIIT involves short bursts of high-intensity exercise followed by periods of rest or low-intensity exercise. This type of exercise can help improve cardiovascular health, manage weight, and improve insulin sensitivity.

Swimming or water aerobics: Swimming or water aerobics can be a low-impact exercise option that is gentle on the joints and can help manage symptoms such as hot flashes and joint pain.

It's important for black women going through menopause to choose exercises that they enjoy and that fit into their lifestyle. Be sure to talk to a healthcare provider before starting any new exercise program.

Eat a healthy diet:

Eating a healthy diet that is rich in fruits, vegetables, whole grains, and lean proteins can help support overall health and manage menopause symptoms.

Foods rich in calcium and vitamin D: Black women are at higher risk for osteoporosis, so it's important to get enough calcium and vitamin D in the diet to support bone health. Good sources of calcium include dairy products and leafy greens. Vitamin D is found in fatty fish, egg yolks, and fortified foods.

Whole grains: Whole grains such as brown rice, quinoa, and oats can help support heart health and manage blood sugar levels.

Lean protein: Lean protein sources such as chicken, fish, beans, and tofu can help support muscle mass and manage weight.

Fruits and vegetables: Fruits and vegetables are rich in vitamins, minerals, and antioxidants that can help support overall health and manage menopause symptoms. Dark leafy greens, berries, citrus fruits, and cruciferous vegetables like broccoli and cauliflower are particularly beneficial.

Healthy fats: Healthy fats such as those found in fatty fish, nuts, seeds, and olive oil can help support heart health and manage inflammation.

Water: Staying hydrated is important during menopause, as it can help manage symptoms such as hot flashes and dry skin. Black women should aim to drink at least 8 cups of water per day.

It's also important to limit or avoid foods that can exacerbate menopause symptoms, such as caffeine, alcohol, spicy foods, and processed foods. Overall, a balanced, nutrient-rich diet can help black women manage their menopause symptoms and support overall health.

Practice stress-reducing techniques:

Stress can exacerbate menopause symptoms, so black women may benefit from practicing stress-reducing techniques such as yoga, meditation, or deep breathing exercises.

Get enough sleep:

Getting enough sleep is important for managing menopause symptoms such as insomnia and fatigue. Black women should aim for 7-8 hours of sleep each night.

Consider hormone therapy:

Hormone therapy can be an effective treatment for menopause symptoms, but it's important to talk to a healthcare provider about the potential risks and benefits.

Seek support:

Joining a support group or talking to friends and family members about menopause can help black women feel less alone and more supported during this transition.

Overall, the experience of menopause among Black women is a complex issue that requires a multifaceted approach. By taking into account the biological, social, and cultural factors that influence the experience of menopause, healthcare providers can work to provide more effective and culturally sensitive care for Black women going through this important life transition.

Vitamins and Supplements Black Women Should Take During Menopause

It's important for black women going through menopause to speak with their healthcare provider before taking any supplements or vitamins. While some supplements may be helpful for managing menopause symptoms, others can interact with medications or have harmful side effects. Here are 10 supplements and vitamins that have been studied for their potential benefits during menopause:

Black cohosh: Black cohosh is an herb that has been used traditionally for menopause symptoms such as hot flashes, mood changes, and sleep disturbances.

Red clover: Red clover is a plant that contains phytoestrogens, which are compounds that can mimic the effects of estrogen in the body. It may be helpful for managing hot flashes and other menopause symptoms.

Vitamin D: Vitamin D is important for bone health and immune function and may also help manage menopause symptoms such as mood changes and joint pain.

Calcium: Calcium is important for bone health, and black women may be at higher risk for osteoporosis, so it's important to get enough calcium in the diet or through supplements.

Menopause and Diversity:

Magnesium: Magnesium is important for muscle and nerve function and may also help manage menopause symptoms such as mood changes and insomnia.

B vitamins: B vitamins, particularly vitamin B6, may be helpful for managing mood changes during menopause.

Omega-3 fatty acids: Omega-3 fatty acids, found in fatty fish and fish oil supplements, may help manage inflammation and support heart health during menopause.

Coenzyme Q10: Coenzyme Q10 is an antioxidant that may help manage hot flashes and other menopause symptoms.

Probiotics: Probiotics may help manage digestive issues and support immune function during menopause.

Melatonin: Melatonin is a hormone that regulates sleep and may be helpful for managing insomnia during menopause.

Asian Women and Menopause

On the other hand, Asian women may have a lower prevalence of menopausal symptoms overall, but they may experience more psychological symptoms such as depression and anxiety.

Again, the reasons for these differences are not fully understood, but some possible explanations have been suggested. For example, cultural attitudes towards menopause may play a role. In some Asian cultures, menopause is viewed as a natural and normal part of the aging process, which may lead to less anxiety and distress surrounding the experience. However, this is a complex issue and cultural attitudes towards menopause can vary widely within and between different Asian cultures.

Asian women experience menopause in diverse ways that are influenced by a variety of factors such as genetics, culture, and lifestyle. While there are similarities in the menopausal experiences of women from different Asian ethnicities, there are also unique differences.

One commonality is that Asian women tend to experience menopause at an earlier age than women from other racial and ethnic groups. This is thought to be due to a combination of genetic and environmental factors. Additionally, Asian women may experience fewer hot flashes compared to women of other races and ethnicities. This may be due in part to the consumption of soy-based foods, which contain natural plant estrogens that can mimic the effects of estrogen in the body.

However, Asian women may also experience unique challenges during menopause, such as an increased risk for osteoporosis. This is because many Asian women have lower bone density compared to women of other races and ethnicities, putting them at greater risk for fractures and other bone-related conditions.

In terms of cultural attitudes and beliefs, menopause is often viewed as a natural and normal part of the aging process in many Asian cultures, and there is less stigma and shame associated with it compared to Western cultures. However, some traditional beliefs may lead to misconceptions and misinformation around menopause, such as the belief that menopause signifies the end of a woman's fertility and femininity.

Furthermore, Asian women may face unique challenges in accessing healthcare and support for menopause-related issues due to language barriers, cultural differences, and a lack of representation and visibility in mainstream healthcare settings. It is important to promote culturally sensitive and inclusive healthcare practices to ensure that all women have access to the support and care they need during menopause.

Bone Density and Asian women

Asian women are known to have lower bone density compared to women of other racial and ethnic groups. This is thought to be due to several factors, including genetics, cultural practices, and lifestyle factors. For example, Asian women tend to have smaller frames and lower body weight compared to women of other ethnicities, which can contribute to lower bone density.

Additionally, traditional cultural practices such as a diet low in calcium and vitamin D, limited exposure to sunlight, and a lack of weight-bearing exercise can also contribute to lower bone density. In some Asian cultures, there is also a preference for consuming foods that are high in oxalates, which can interfere with calcium absorption and contribute to lower bone density.

Low bone density puts Asian women at greater risk for osteoporosis, a condition in which the bones become weak and brittle and are more prone to fractures. Osteoporosis is a significant health concern for women in menopause, as the drop in estrogen levels during this time can further exacerbate bone loss.

It is important for Asian women to prioritize bone health during menopause by consuming a diet rich in calcium and vitamin D, doing regular weight-bearing exercise, and limiting alcohol and smoking, both of which can contribute to bone loss. It is also important for women to discuss their risk for osteoporosis with their healthcare provider and consider bone density screening and appropriate interventions such as calcium and vitamin D supplements or medication if necessary.

Menopause and Diversity:

Depression and Anxiety in Asian Women in Menopause

Depression and anxiety are common psychological symptoms experienced by women during menopause, including Asian women. The changes in hormonal levels during menopause can contribute to mood fluctuations, which can lead to feelings of sadness, irritability, and anxiety. Additionally, cultural and social factors can also impact the experience of depression and anxiety in Asian women.

In some Asian cultures, there is a strong emphasis on stoicism and emotional restraint, this means that people are expected to keep their emotions in check and not display them openly. This can make it difficult for Asian women going through menopause to express their emotions and seek help for psychological symptoms like depression and anxiety.

In many Asian cultures, mental health is still stigmatized, and seeking help for emotional struggles is often seen as a sign of weakness. Moreover, the concept of saving face is also important in some Asian cultures, which can make it challenging for women to admit to having mental health struggles and seek help for fear of being seen as a burden on their families or community. This can make it challenging for Asian women to express their emotional struggles and seek help and can contribute to feelings of isolation and worsen symptoms of depression and anxiety.

It is important for Asian women to be aware of the signs and symptoms of depression and anxiety during menopause and to seek help from healthcare professionals or mental health specialists if necessary. Seeking support from family members and community resources can also be helpful in managing these symptoms. Additionally, healthcare providers should be aware of cultural factors that may impact the experience of depression and anxiety in Asian women and provide culturally sensitive care.

Family Responsibilities and Caregiver Duties of The Asian Woman

Family responsibilities, caregiving duties, and cultural expectations around aging can also contribute to increased stress and emotional burden for Asian women during menopause. In many Asian cultures, women are expected to prioritize the needs of their families over their own. This expectation can lead to women neglecting their own health, including their menopausal symptoms, in order to fulfill their familial obligations. For example, some Asian women may not seek medical help for their menopausal symptoms because they do not want to burden their families with the additional financial or time costs of seeking medical care.

Additionally, family dynamics may change during menopause as women experience physical and emotional changes. Women may feel pressure to maintain their role as caregivers and continue to fulfill their familial responsibilities, even as they experience symptoms like hot flashes, mood swings, and fatigue.

However, it is important for women to prioritize their own health and well-being during menopause. Neglecting menopausal symptoms can have negative long-term effects on women's health, including increased risk for osteoporosis, cardiovascular disease, and other health issues. It is important for women to communicate their needs to their families and seek support from their loved ones to help manage their symptoms and prioritize their health.

Furthermore, healthcare providers should be aware of the cultural and social expectations around family responsibility in Asian communities and provide culturally sensitive care. This can include discussing the importance of self-care and the impact that menopausal symptoms can have on women's health and quality of life. Providing education and resources to women and their families can also help them navigate the challenges of menopause while maintaining their familial responsibilities.

Healthcare For the Asian Woman During Menopause

Accessing healthcare during menopause can be challenging for Asian women due to various cultural, linguistic, and socioeconomic factors. In many Asian cultures, discussing personal health concerns is considered taboo, and seeking medical help may be seen as a sign of weakness. Additionally, language barriers and limited access to healthcare services can make it difficult for some Asian women to receive proper care.

Another issue is the lack of awareness and education about menopause among Asian women. Many women may not understand the changes that are occurring in their bodies and may not realize that the symptoms they are experiencing are related to menopause. This can lead to underreporting of symptoms and delays in seeking medical care.

Furthermore, socioeconomic factors such as limited health insurance coverage and financial constraints may prevent some Asian women from seeking medical help for their menopausal symptoms.

To address these challenges, healthcare providers should be aware of the unique needs and challenges faced by Asian women during menopause. Culturally sensitive care, including providing education and resources in a culturally appropriate manner, can help increase awareness about menopause and encourage women to seek medical help when needed. This may include working with community organizations to provide outreach and education to Asian women, as well as offering language interpretation services and ensuring access to affordable healthcare services.

Things Asian Women Can Do to Help with Their Symptoms of Menopause

Asian women going through menopause can benefit from a range of lifestyle changes and natural remedies to help manage symptoms. Here are some things that may be helpful:

Incorporate soy into the diet: Soy contains phytoestrogens, which are plant compounds that can mimic the effects of estrogen in the body. Soy foods such as tofu, tempeh, and edamame may help manage hot flashes and other menopause symptoms.

Eat a balanced diet: A balanced diet that is rich in fruits, vegetables, whole grains, lean protein, and healthy fats can help support overall health and manage symptoms such as weight gain and fatigue.

Get regular exercise: Regular exercise, such as brisk walking, yoga, or tai chi, can help manage mood changes, improve sleep, and support overall health.

Practice stress-reducing techniques: Stress can exacerbate menopause symptoms, so it's important to find ways to manage stress such as meditation, deep breathing, or acupuncture.

Use natural remedies: Certain natural remedies may be helpful for managing menopause symptoms, such as black cohosh, red clover, and dong quai. However, it's important to talk to a healthcare provider before using any natural remedies, as they may interact with medications or have harmful side effects.

Stay hydrated: Drinking plenty of water and avoiding caffeine and alcohol can help manage hot flashes and other menopause symptoms.

Get enough sleep: Good quality sleep is important for managing menopause symptoms such as fatigue and mood changes. Establishing a regular sleep routine and avoiding stimulants such as caffeine and electronic devices before bed can help improve sleep quality.

Asian Women and Menopause

As with any supplement, it's important for Asian women to talk to their healthcare provider before taking any new supplements during menopause. That being said, here are some supplements that may be helpful for managing menopause symptoms in Asian women:

Black cohosh: Black cohosh is an herb that has been traditionally used to manage menopause symptoms such as hot flashes, mood changes, and sleep disturbances.

Soy isoflavones: Soy isoflavones are plant compounds that can mimic the effects of estrogen in the body. They may be helpful for managing hot flashes and other menopause symptoms in Asian women.

Vitamin D: Vitamin D is important for bone health and immune function and may also help manage menopause symptoms such as mood changes and joint pain.

Calcium: Calcium is important for bone health, and Asian women may be at higher risk for osteoporosis, so it's important to get enough calcium in the diet or through supplements.

Magnesium: Magnesium is important for muscle and nerve function and may also help manage menopause symptoms such as mood changes and insomnia.

B vitamins: B vitamins, particularly vitamin B6, may be helpful for managing mood changes during menopause.

Omega-3 fatty acids: Omega-3 fatty acids, found in fatty fish and fish oil supplements, may help manage inflammation and support heart health during menopause.

.

Again, it's important for Asian women going through menopause to talk to a healthcare provider about the best strategies for managing their symptoms based on their individual needs and health history.

European Women and Menopause

European women experience menopause like women from other regions, with a gradual decrease in ovarian function and estrogen production. However, studies have shown that European women may have some unique characteristics related to menopause. Here are some of the key things' women should know about menopause in European women:

Age at menopause:

The average age at which European women experience menopause is around 51, which is similar to the age of women in other regions such as North America and Australia.

Hot flashes:

Hot flashes are a common symptom of menopause, and studies have shown that European women tend to have a higher prevalence of hot flashes than women from other regions such as Asia and Africa.

Hormone replacement therapy (HRT):

HRT is a treatment option for menopausal symptoms, and studies have shown that European women have higher rates of HRT use than women from other regions. However, rates of

HRT use vary widely across European countries, with higher rates in northern and western European countries and lower rates in southern and eastern European countries.

Osteoporosis:

Osteoporosis is a common condition in postmenopausal women, and studies have shown that European women have a higher risk of osteoporosis than women from other regions. This may be due in part to differences in lifestyle factors such as diet and physical activity.

Mental health:

Menopause can also have an impact on women's mental health, and studies have shown that European women may be at higher risk for depression and anxiety during the menopausal transition than women from other regions.

It's important to remember that each woman's experience of menopause is unique, and factors such as lifestyle, genetics, and healthcare access can all play a role in how menopause is experienced. If you're experiencing menopausal symptoms, talk to your healthcare provider about options for managing them.

Menopause and Diversity:

Indigenous Women and Menopause

Indigenous women have been shown to experience menopause earlier and have a higher risk of certain health conditions associated with menopause compared to other racial groups.

Studies have shown that Indigenous women tend to experience menopause earlier than other racial groups, with an average age of onset between 46 and 48 years old. They also tend to have higher rates of hot flashes, night sweats, and other menopausal symptoms.

In addition, Indigenous women may be at higher risk for certain health conditions associated with menopause, including cardiovascular disease, osteoporosis, and depression. This may be due to a combination of genetic, environmental, and lifestyle factors.

Early onset of menopause:

Studies have shown that Indigenous women tend to experience menopause at an earlier age than other racial groups. This can be due to a combination of genetic, environmental, and lifestyle factors, including higher rates of smoking and exposure to environmental toxins.

Increased risk of certain health conditions:

Indigenous women may be at higher risk for certain health conditions associated with menopause, including cardiovascular disease, osteoporosis, and depression. This may be due to a combination of factors, including genetic predisposition, lifestyle factors such as diet and physical activity, and social determinants of health such as poverty and discrimination. Menopause can also have an impact on Indigenous women's mental health. Studies have shown that Indigenous women may be at higher risk for depression and anxiety during the menopausal transition, which can be linked to a range of factors including social isolation, loss of cultural roles and responsibilities, and the impact of historical trauma.

Lack of access to healthcare:

Indigenous women may face barriers to accessing healthcare and support during the menopausal transition. This can include a lack of culturally appropriate healthcare services, geographic barriers to healthcare access, and financial barriers to accessing care.

Traditional healing practices:

Indigenous women may also rely on traditional healing practices to manage menopausal symptoms. These practices can include the use of herbal remedies, traditional medicines, and cultural practices such as ceremony and prayer. Traditional healing practices and medicines can play an important role in supporting Indigenous women's health and well-being during the menopausal transition. For example, some Indigenous cultures use plants such as black cohosh, red clover, and sage to manage menopausal symptoms

Cultural factors:

Menopause may also be viewed differently in Indigenous cultures, with some cultures viewing it as a time of wisdom and spiritual transformation. However, there can also be stigma and taboo around menopause, which can make it difficult for women to seek help and support for their symptoms. Menopause can have a significant impact on Indigenous women's cultural roles and responsibilities. For example, in some Indigenous cultures, menopause marks a shift in a woman's role from caregiver to mentor, and women may be expected to take on new roles and responsibilities within their communities. Indigenous women come from diverse cultural backgrounds and may have different beliefs, attitudes, and practices related to menopause. For example, some Indigenous cultures view menopause as a time of spiritual transformation, while others may view it more negatively. Understanding and respecting these cultural differences is important for providing culturally sensitive healthcare services and support.

Geographic location:

Indigenous women living in rural and remote communities may face additional challenges during the menopausal transition. They may have limited access to healthcare services, including gynecological care and menopause management resources. This can make it difficult for them to receive the care and support they need to manage symptoms and maintain their health.

It's important for Indigenous women to have access to culturally appropriate healthcare and support during the menopausal transition. This can include education about menopause and its associated health risks, as well as access to treatments and therapies that can help manage symptoms and reduce the risk of complications. Culturally sensitive healthcare services that integrate traditional healing practices can also play an important role in supporting Indigenous women's health and well-being during the menopausal transition.

It's important for Indigenous women to have access to culturally appropriate healthcare and support during the menopausal transition. This can include education about menopause and its associated health risks, as well as access to treatments and therapies that can help manage symptoms and reduce the risk of complications. Also understanding the demographic factors that impact Indigenous women's experience of menopause is important for providing appropriate and effective healthcare services and support. This can help ensure that Indigenous women receive the care and support they need to manage symptoms and maintain their health and well-being during this life transition.

Menopause and Diversity:

Things Indigenous Women Can do During Menopause

Indigenous women may face unique challenges when it comes to managing menopause symptoms, due to factors such as cultural differences, historical trauma, and lack of access to healthcare resources. Here are some things that Indigenous women may want to consider when managing menopause.

Seek out traditional healing practices: Many Indigenous cultures have traditional healing practices that may be helpful for managing menopause symptoms, such as herbal remedies, smudging, and spiritual practices. Indigenous women may want to consider incorporating these practices into their menopause management plan.

Connect with other Indigenous women: Menopause can be an isolating experience, and connecting with other Indigenous women going through menopause can provide a sense of community and support. Indigenous women may want to consider joining a menopause support group or connecting with other women through social media or other online platforms.

Address historical trauma: Indigenous women may be dealing with intergenerational trauma related to colonization and other historical traumas. Addressing these issues through counseling or therapy may be helpful for managing menopause symptoms.

Address healthcare disparities: Indigenous women may face healthcare disparities that make it more difficult to access healthcare resources. It's important for Indigenous women to advocate for themselves and seek out healthcare resources that are culturally sensitive and address their unique needs of Indigenous women. This may involve doing some research and asking for recommendations from other Indigenous women.

Advocate for themselves and their healthcare needs. Indigenous women may need to be assertive and speak up for themselves to ensure that they are receiving the care that they need.

Connect with community organizations and resources that can provide support and information about healthcare resources that are available to Indigenous women.

Work to address systemic issues that contribute to healthcare disparities, such as lack of funding for Indigenous healthcare programs and lack of access to healthcare resources in Indigenous communities.

Manage stress: Stress can exacerbate menopause symptoms, so managing stress is an important part of menopause management. Indigenous women may want to consider traditional stress management practices such as meditation, yoga, or mindfulness.

Again, it's important for Indigenous women to talk to their healthcare provider about the best strategies for managing their menopause symptoms based on their individual needs and health history.

Lifestyle Factors

Lifestyle factors can play a significant role in the experience of menopause for all women, regardless of race or ethnicity. Here are some ways in which lifestyle can affect menopause:

Diet:

A healthy diet is important for all women during menopause. Eating a balanced diet rich in fruits, vegetables, whole grains, and lean protein can help maintain a healthy weight, reduce the risk of chronic diseases, and support bone health. Some studies have also suggested that certain foods or supplements, such as soy or black cohosh, may help alleviate menopausal symptoms, although more research is needed.

Exercise:

Regular exercise has been shown to have numerous benefits for menopausal women, including improved mood, reduced hot flashes, and better bone health. Women are encouraged to engage in moderate-intensity aerobic exercise, such as brisk walking or cycling, for at least 150 minutes per week, as well as strength training exercises to maintain muscle mass and bone density.

Smoking:

Smoking can increase the risk of numerous health problems, including heart disease, osteoporosis, and certain cancers, all of which may be of particular concern for menopausal women. Smoking cessation is strongly recommended for all women, but especially for those going through menopause.

Alcohol consumption:

Excessive alcohol consumption can increase the risk of breast cancer and other health problems and may exacerbate menopausal symptoms such as hot flashes and sleep disturbances. Women are advised to limit their alcohol intake to no more than one drink per day.

Stress management:

Menopause can be a stressful time for many women, and chronic stress can have negative effects on health and well-being. Women are encouraged to develop stress-management techniques, such as meditation, yoga, or counseling, to help cope with the challenges of menopause.

Sleep:

Getting adequate sleep is important for overall health and can be particularly challenging for menopausal women who may experience sleep disturbances such as hot flashes or night sweats. Women are advised to practice good sleep hygiene, such as maintaining a regular sleep schedule, creating a comfortable sleep environment, and avoiding caffeine and alcohol before bedtime.

Sexual health:

Menopause can affect women's sexual health in numerous ways, including vaginal dryness, decreased libido, and pain during intercourse. Women are encouraged to discuss any concerns with their healthcare provider and explore treatment options such as lubricants, hormone therapy, or other medications.

It's important to note that lifestyle factors can interact with other factors, such as genetics, medical history, and cultural attitudes, to influence the experience of menopause. Women are encouraged to work with their healthcare providers to develop a personalized plan for managing menopause symptoms and maintaining optimal health and well-being.

Socioeconomic Status and Menopause

Socioeconomic status can play a significant role in how women experience menopause. Women with lower socioeconomic status (SES) may experience more severe menopausal symptoms and have limited access to healthcare, which can make managing menopause more challenging.

There are several ways that SES can affect menopause:

Access to healthcare:

Women with lower SES may have limited access to healthcare, which can make managing menopause more difficult. For example, they may be less likely to receive regular gynecological exams or have access to hormone replacement therapy (HRT), which can help alleviate some menopausal symptoms. Rich people are more likely to have access to high-quality healthcare services, including gynecological care and menopause management resources. They may be able to afford regular check-ups and screenings and have access to a range of treatments and therapies to manage menopausal symptoms. Poor people, on the other hand, may face barriers to accessing healthcare services, including lack of health insurance or financial resources to pay for care.

Menopause and Diversity:

Stress:

Women with lower SES may experience more stress in their daily lives, which can exacerbate menopausal symptoms. Chronic stress has been linked to hot flashes, night sweats, and mood changes, all of which are common symptoms of menopause.

Lifestyle factors:

Women with lower SES may be more likely to smoke, drink alcohol, and have a poor diet, which can worsen menopausal symptoms. Rich people may be more likely to have access to healthy foods, exercise facilities, and other resources that can help them manage menopausal symptoms. Poor people, on the other hand, may face challenges in maintaining a healthy lifestyle, such as limited access to healthy food options or safe spaces to exercise.

Work environment:

Women with lower SES may work in jobs that are physically demanding or have long hours, which can make managing menopausal symptoms challenging. Rich people may have more flexibility in their work and caregiving responsibilities, which can make it easier to manage menopausal symptoms. For example, they may be able to take time off from work or hire help with caregiving responsibilities if needed. Poor people, on the other hand, may have less flexibility in their work and caregiving responsibilities, which can make it difficult to manage menopausal symptoms and maintain their health.

Education level:

Women with lower SES may have lower levels of education, which can affect their knowledge about menopause and available treatments. This can make it more difficult for them to manage symptoms effectively.

Support:

Rich people may have more access to social support networks, including friends, family members, and support groups, which can help them manage menopausal symptoms. Poor people, on the other hand, may have limited social support networks, which can make it difficult to manage symptoms and maintain their mental and emotional health.

It's important to note that women with lower SES are not the only ones who experience menopausal symptoms. However, the impact of SES on menopause underscores the importance of access to healthcare and education about menopause for all women, regardless of socioeconomic status. If you're experiencing menopausal symptoms, talk to your healthcare provider about options for managing them.

SUMMARY

Menopause affects women of different races and ethnicities in unique ways due to biological, cultural, and socioeconomic factors. For example, Black women may experience more severe symptoms due to differences in hormone levels and increased stress related to systemic racism. Asian women may experience hot flashes less frequently but may be more susceptible to osteoporosis. Indigenous women may experience cultural and historical trauma that can impact their menopause experience and access to healthcare resources.

To manage menopause symptoms, women of different races can take a variety of approaches, including dietary changes, exercise, stress management techniques, and supplements. It is also important to seek out culturally sensitive healthcare providers who understand the unique needs of women from diverse backgrounds. Addressing healthcare disparities, which can impact access to care and treatment outcomes, is also crucial for women from marginalized communities. By taking a holistic approach and addressing the unique factors that impact menopause for women of different races and ethnicities, women can successfully manage their symptoms and maintain their health and well-being throughout this important life stage.

REFERENCES

Menopause Symptoms Are Worse For Black Women, But They're Less Likely to Receive Medical Help | HuffPost UK Life (huffingtonpost.co.uk)

2. Racial and Ethnic Disparities in Menopause | Everyday Health
3. Duration of the menopausal transition is longer in women with young age at onset: the multi- ethnic Study of Women's Health Across the Nation - PMC (nih.gov)
4. What Is Vaginal Dryness? Symptoms, Causes, Diagnosis, Treatment, and Prevention | Everyday HealthHow Race Affects Menopause | MenoLabs
5. How Race Affects Menopause | MenoLabs

www.ingramcontent.com/pod-product-compliance
Lightning Source LLC
Chambersburg PA
CBHW070036040426
42333CB00040B/1696